Updated Paleo Diet Food List

by

Rachel Hathaway

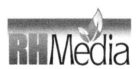

Updated Paleo Diet Food List

ISBN-13: 978-1499611984

ISBN-10: 1499611986

are assumed to be the property of their respective owners, and are used only for reference. There is no implied endorsement if we use one of these terms. Finally, use your own judgement. Nothing in this ebook/guide is intended to replace common sense, legal, medical, or other professional advice, and is meant only to inform and entertain the reader.

Updated Paleo Diet Food List

Introduction

Thanks for checking out my new book!

When my Mom, who has tried every diet under the sun, told me that she was switching to a Paleo Diet and having some early success, I immediately asked her what she can eat.

I thought it was a simple question.

I guess I was wrong...

She had a vague answer about "hunter/gatherers" and how it was probably the very first human diet. She said she had heard that the diet of most Americans/ Europeans consists of about 70% processed foods. But when it came right down to it, she wasn't all that sure about the specifics of the plan.

After telling me some weird story about old stone tools, and then digressing about the weather in her part of the country, she mentioned a few recipes books that she had tried and started rattling off some of the ingredients in those.

"Not super helpful, Mom."

"Why?" she asked.

So I told her, "Mom, this is what I need: I need an absolutely useable food list for a Paleo diet!"

And, more importantly, I wanted to know which foods to avoid.

I wanted to know straight away, not through a series of disconnected recipes...

And then after doing a bunch of research with the staffers at RH Media, we came up with this newly UPDATED PALEO FOOD LIST, and the very first copy will go to my Mom!

(Let's call it a late/early Mother's Day gift!)

Why?

It's fine to follow a new (old) diet, especially one that seems to be working for you, but recipes can be sort of limiting.

I want to know what to buy, what I should eat when I'm at home, and what I'm able to eat when I go to a restaurant. I need to plan meals for the week, or I won't really stick to ANY plan. I know myself too well. I have shelves of great recipe books, and the photos are spectacular, but I can count on one hand how many of those recipes I've made.

I can't constantly cross-reference Paleo diet breakfast, lunch, and dinner recipes to build a series of meals, especially my lunches for work. I want to have a good idea now of what's likely IN and what's OUT with this diet.

And when I see online that Paleo can still work vegan at times (we try once a week), and I can still fire up the slow cooker, I want to know how.

WHAT THIS BOOK IS AND WHAT IT ISN'T

First of all, this book is not some blanket endorsement of a Paleo diet. I'm not really sure how well it works YET, and whatever I've heard is just chatter among some of my peeps.

Enough said.

So that means you need to make up your own mind if a Paleo diet plan even makes sense for you. (You should probably also consult your doctor or other medical professional before you make changes to your diet anyway. That's what I try to do.) I don't know if I'll lose weight, look great in my bathing suit, or have a lot more energy, but I do know I need this list!!

After that, please understand that there are no recipes here. This is a book about possibilities, and actually helps me more than flipping through a number of possibly tasty recipes, all the while keeping an eye on the estimated PREP time. Personally, I look down these lists here and see hundreds of recipes between the lines.

I just want a PALEO FOOD LIST to have a quick look at the ingredients that I should watch for at the store, and, according to this plan, things I should probably skip. And since I can have this ebook on my smartphone, problem solved!

Simple, huh?

That's the beauty of this. Hopefully, you'll agree.

So let's get started.

CHAPTER ONE

Fresh Fruits & Vegetables

So when it comes to vegetables in a Paleo diet, you're pretty much smooth sailing. This is why it's still totally possible to have our once-a-week vegan nights. The only thing to watch out for is legumes, starchy vegetables like potatoes, and high-sugar fruits like bananas, which aren't that good for you on any diet plan.

If you keep an eye out for some of these fruits and veggies on your next shopping trip, you can add a lot of great new flavors to your menus. (I made a point to get some cauliflower, a mango, and a bag of limes on a recent outing, and added some real variety to our week!) So here you go:

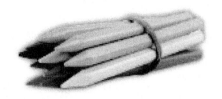

PALEO FRUIT & VEGETABLE LIST

Apples
Apricots
Artichoke Hearts
Asparagus
Avocadoes
Bananas (in moderation)
Beets
Blackberries
Blueberries
Broccoli
Brussel Sprouts
Cabbage
Cantaloupe
Carrots
Cauliflower
Celery
Cherries
Collard Greens
Cranberries
Cucumber
Eggplant
Endive
Figs

Grapefruit
Grapes
Green Onions
Guava
Kale
Kiwi
Lemons
Limes
Lychee
Mangoes
Mushrooms
Mustard Greens
Olives
Oranges
Papaya
Parsley
Parsnip
Passion Fruit
Peaches
Pears
Peppers (red, green, yellow)
Persimmon
Pineapple
Plums
Pomegranate
Pumpkin
Raspberries
Romaine Lettuce
Rhubarb
Rutabaga
Seaweed (kelp)

Snow Peas
Spinach
Sprouts
Squash
Star Fruit
Strawberries
Swiss Chard
Tangerines
Turnips
Watercress
Watermelon
Zucchini

As with many other contemporary diets, raw fruits and vegetables are pretty good for your overall energy level. I also like to drop a bunch of these fruits and veggies together into my blender/juicer machine and try to make a WOWSER drink in the morning, but raw is still the best! (Yes, I use "wowser" as a sort of technical term for really good, just go with it.)

With the right blender-bullet thingy (you know the one!), we can also grind up all of the skins, nuts, and oils we want as well. I feel better about this process than what we did with our old juicer, where it felt we were wasting so many nutritional parts of the fruits and veggies. (We've recently made some crazy-fun PALEO smoothies for example with plums, strawberries, a little spinach, a spot of olive oil, and some pumpkin seeds... it's actually really delicious as long as you use enough strawberries!)

So, as I told my Mom (and everyone else in my world!), this raw fruits/veggies thing is, OF COURSE, the perfect argument for buying organically grown fruits and veggies. Sure they wash everything, we wash everything (twice!), but if you're going to be chomping on raw stuff, isn't it better to know that it didn't have any artificial pesticides on them at any point?

We think it's totally worth it to buy organic, and since every store seems to be getting on the bandwagon of increased food safety, it's easier to find a huge variety of stuff. Plus if we all buy organic, which was the old-fashioned way before they invented all of these crazy pesticides, then the prices will have to come down. OK, Mom, I'll get off my soap box.

Next, to the meat category...

CHAPTER TWO

Meats

Of course with a Paleo diet you need to stay away from processed meats like salami, bologna, hot dogs, and other deli wonders, but that still leaves room for a lot of other choices.

A lot. Quite.

Because of the nature of the Paleolithic diet though, a fair amount of the things you can eat in the meat category are downright strange and impractical. My Mom and her (third) husband live in the South so maybe they can find some of this stuff (doubt it!), but in New England my sweetie and I wouldn't even know where to start.

Be on the lookout for grass-fed and/or free range meat by the way, which is what you usually get when you ask for organic meat. It might take an extra detour on your way home from work, but it's worth it. (The image on our book cover is also a subtle reminder...)

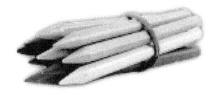

PALEO MEAT LIST

Bacon (in moderation)
Bear
Beef Jerky
Bison
Bison Jerky
Bison Ribeye
Bison Sirloin
Bison Steaks
Buffalo
Chicken Breast (free range)
Chicken Thighs (free range)
Chuck Steak
Elk
Emu
Goat
Goose
Ground Beef (free range)
Kangaroo
Lamb Rack
Lean Veal
New York Steak

Ostrich
Pheasant
Poultry (above)
Pork
Pork Chops
Pork Tenderloin
Quail
Rabbit
Rattlesnake
Reindeer
Steak (above)
Turkey
Turtle
Veal
Venison Steaks
Wild Boar

Ok, seriously I can't imagine eating bear, emu, kangaroo, ostrich, or rattlesnake, but that's me. I get a little snooty when the WIFI is down for more than fifteen minutes, so just thinking about those "meats" makes me feel WAY too rustic. And as for reindeer, I can't go there either. Too many holiday decorations bouncing around in my head, I guess. But after getting this all together, now I know why people keep mentioning bison burgers.

If you simply choose one to start with ~ like turkey, for example ~ you'll find that you're approach to preparing the meals is too limited. Forget about a single favorite recipe, family expectations, or any of that. Start from scratch. Look at these ingredients and think about the range of amazing ways you can prepare dinners for your table.

I take the same approach with everything on this list -- within reason. It's lead me to reevaluate the way we prepare beef, pork, veal, steak, and more.

But now you know the full monty, Mom (and all my other wonderful readers)! But seriously, good luck finding wild boar at your local deli or supermarket.

So, let's take a look at the fish and seafood list now...

CHAPTER THREE

Fish & Seafood

Fish and a wide range of seafood and shellfish are abundant on the Paleo list. That's good because of the protein and the magic of Omega 3's. We were very happy to discover a collection of easy to find, tasty fresh and salt-water fish, and enough other choices for those special occasions.

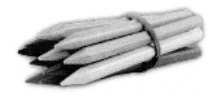

PALEO FISH & SEAFOOD LIST

Bass
Clams
Crab
Crawfish

Crayfish
Halibut
Lobster
Mackerel
Oysters
Red Snapper
Salmon
Sardines
Scallops
Shark
Shrimp
Sole
Sunfish
Swordfish
Tilapia
Trout
Tuna
Wallete

For me, this list has been very helpful when we go out to eat. Swordfish, cooked in olive oil, served with lemon and garnished with parsley was something I was able to get on our last trip into the big city. (Protein and vegetables, low salt ~ that's always my restaurant plan these days.)

That was my first attempt to see how possible it was to follow a Paleo diet on the go!

Nailed it. (But, I'm not trying shark, though. Ever.)

Eggs are up next.

CHAPTER FOUR

Eggs

For eggs, I was glad to know that they're on the list.

What to look for:

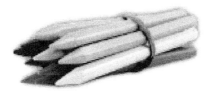

PALEO EGG LIST

Chicken eggs
Duck eggs
Goose eggs

If you can find a local farm and get some of these as free range, pastured, or organic, it's always worth it because I think the eggs are just plain better. The large goose and duck eggs are a must-have in our household now.

Pretty straightforward, huh.

Next up...

CHAPTER FIVE

Nuts & Seeds

I love nuts, seeds, and all manner of trail mix. After ditching processed foods, trail mix has become our snack of choice.

But honestly I had always been suspicious of nuts and seeds because they tasted so good. I know they have lots of protein, BUT they can also be high in fat.

Paleo diets suggest skipping peanuts (a legume, right!) and cashews, but the rest of these should really make for tasty snacks, and don't forget to use them as integral cooking ingredients.

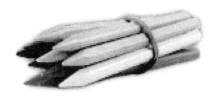

PALEO NUTS & SEEDS LIST

Almonds
Cashews
Hazelnuts
Macadamia Nuts
Pecans
Pine Nuts
Pumpkin Seeds
Sunflower Seeds
Walnuts

Of course, when I purchase these, I always look for the unsalted variety.

Next up, this brings us to healthy oils...

CHAPTER SIX

Healthy Oils & Fats

I still haven't been able to find the first one on this oils list, but I'm still looking!

This is a list of healthy oils and fats that shows up on almost everyone's "USE INSTEAD" lists! It's funny that Paleo confirms many of the things we see elsewhere about these oils.

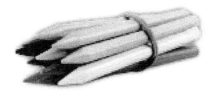

PALEO HEALTHY OILS & FATS LIST

Avocado Oil
Butter (grass fed)
Coconut Oil

Macadamia Oil
Olive Oil

Our staff found online that there's an interesting connection to this type of diet, without salt and processed foods, to acne. High protein diets with these oils are apparently reopening studies around the globe of connections between diet and acne, since the skin reflects what's going on in the body.

That's cool, although I'm way past my acne years... that ship has sailed.

NEXT UP:

The long-awaited "foods I should not eat, seriously avoid, or at least handle with care on my Paleo-inspired diet..."

CHAPTER SEVEN

Food to Avoid on a Paleo Diet

If you need an ANTI-SHOPPING grocery list for your Paleo diet, here it is.

I asked my Mom what stuff I should NOT buy at all of the very cool food stores near where I live, and she was stumped. Coming up with this info seems to be the most perplexing part for most new people on the Paleo diet.

As I mentioned before, this is a combination DO NOT EAT, TRY TO AVOID, or at least HANDLE WITH CARE list. In the real world, having an english muffin isn't grounds for a court-martial.

But to get the full impact of a Paleo-inspired diet, don't plan on eating or drinking these items:

PALEO AVOID LIST

Acorn squash

Beans (adzuki, black, broad, fava, garbanzo, green, kidney, lima, mung, navy, pinto, red, string, white)

Beer or hard alcohol

Beets

Bread/Toast

Butter (unless it's grass fed)

Butternut squash

Candy/junk food

Cereal Grains

Cheese

Corn

Corn syrup

Cottage Cheese

Crackers

Cream Cheese

Doughnuts

English Muffins

Hash Browns

High Sugar/Fructose Fruit Juices (apple, chinola, grape, mango, orange, starfruit, or strawberry)

Hot Dogs

Ice Cream

Ice Milk

French Fries

Frozen Yogurt

Ketchup

Legumes

Lentils

Milk (skim, 2%, low fat, or whole milk)

Miso

Non-fat Dairy Creamer
Oatmeal
Pancakes
Pasta (all types including lasagna, spaghetti, rigatoni, and fettuccini)
Peas (black-eyed, chickpeas, snow peas, snap peas)
Peanuts
Peanut Butter
Potatoes
Powdered Milk
Processed Foods (chips, cookies, pastries, or pretzels)
Refined Sugar (and artificial sweeteners)
Reined Vegetable Oils
Salt
Soda or Energy Drinks
Soybeans (and soybean products)
Spam
Sweet Potatoes
Wheat
Yams
Yogurt
Yucca

Of course, I could have listed SEVERAL hundred brand-name products by name, but I figure you get the idea. Much of our cabinets were overflowing with all manner of cookies, snacks, pretzels, and chips. Candy is obvious, and we made a deal to finish the ice cream in the freezer before we adopted the plan. (I don't like to waste food!)

I understand it may take some serious changes for you to enforce this type of list, but if we can manage it in our house, yours should be a SNAP!

CHAPTER EIGHT

Paleo Diet Food Shopping List Samples

So those lists should help you at the grocery store, but I put together a few specific shopping lists that might inspire you to eat better. Again, since there aren't any recipes here, this is about seeing the possibilities in a list of wonderful, fresh, raw ingredients. I tend to improvise in the kitchen anyway. (I must have been a jazz singer in a past life!)

And as I mentioned before, try to find as many of these as you can in their USDA certified organic varieties. I think they taste better and we're still going for critical mass on lowering the cost, folks!

So let's take a look:

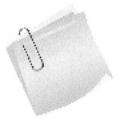

SAMPLE PALEO SHOPPING LIST - Number One

Green Apples (organic)
Celery (organic)
Avocado (organic)
Eggplant (organic)
Green Onions (organic)
Coconut Oil
Free-range Chicken Thighs/Breasts
New York Steak
Fresh Tuna
Walnuts
Chicken Eggs (free range; organic)

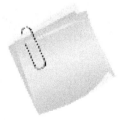

SAMPLE PALEO SHOPPING LIST - Number Two

Artichoke hearts (organic)
Cabbage (organic)
Carrots (organic)
Cherries (organic)
Peaches (organic)
Red and Yellow Peppers (organic)
Olive Oil (organic)
Pork Tenderloin
Ground beef (free range)
Chicken Breast (free range)
Lean Veal
Halibut
Shrimp
Pumpkin Seeds
Pecans
Duck or Goose Eggs (free range; organic)

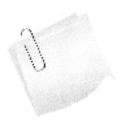

SAMPLE PALEO SHOPPING LIST - Number Three

Blueberries (organic)
Grapes (organic)
Oranges (organic)
Spinach (organic)

Cauliflower (organic)
Green Peppers (organic)
Parsley (organic)
Zucchini (organic)
Avocado Oil (organic)
Pork Chops
Beef Jerky
Bison Steaks
Chicken Thighs (free range)
Turkey
Crab
Scallops
Lobster
Hazelnuts
Sunflower Seeds
Pine Nuts
Duck or Goose Eggs (free range; organic)

***

I hope these sample shopping lists inspire you to become a better, healthier shopper starting with your next trip to the store. Be creative, be open-minded, and consider buying ingredients to just cook and combine in interesting ways at home. And if you find some great Paleo recipes, then by all means use them. (But don't be afraid to make some creative substitutions using this guide!)

CHAPTER NINE

Closing Thoughts

I hope this book has been helpful.

Are you really surprised that we feel the way we do? I know I eat like crap, my sweet-heart eats like crap (as much as I do), our little cherub eats like crap when it's up to her, and most people I know battle with this too.

The typical modern American diet has seriously been on the MUST-CHANGE path for a while!

It's interesting that this "modern" change to Paleo is basically a major flashback to a "hunter-gatherer" diet which was all the rage 10,000+ years ago.

Do you need more clues here about removing salt and processed foods from your diet, already knowing that it's clearly a dangerous part of your regular intake? I don't.

(Makes me wonder what else they knew 10,000+ years ago that we should check out!) I guess we have the best of both worlds. Their streamlined diet and my high-speed internet...

But before I wrap this up, let me tell you about our changes:

We have tried to back off on the grains, avoid sugar and corn syrup entirely, and eat fresh raw fruits and veggies all throughout the day. (Can I tell you how much I love local farmers' markets!) And we're almost always cooking now with coconut oil. I'll let you know if I lose any weight, but for now I feel inspired.

I seriously hope you enjoyed this brief ebook of lists, and that it helps you plan better shopping trips AND partake in healthier eating at restaurants. (Plus it makes a nice gift for my Mom, and all her friends)!

Good luck finding those crazy meats, BTW! And bon appetite.

CHAPTER TEN

Did You Like: Updated Paleo Diet Food List

If you enjoyed reading this book, I would love it if you would help others enjoy it as well. **LEND** it, **RECOMMEND** it, or **REVIEW** it.

You can share it with a friend via the lending feature, which has been enabled for this book. Or you can help other readers find this book by recommending it to friends and family, reading and discussion groups, online forums, or other sites. You can also review it on the site where you purchased it. If you do happen to write a review, please inform me via an email to rachelhathawaywriter@gmail.com, and I'll thank you with a personal email.

Links to my other titles can be found here:

http://www.amazon.com/Rachel-Hathaway/e/B00KFFLX10

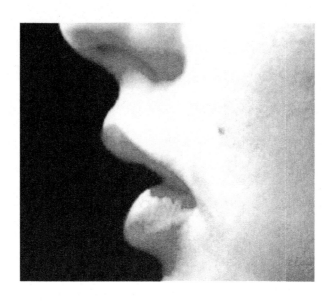

Rachel Hathaway is the pen name for a professional writer whom you may or may not know (Mysterious, huh?). Her work spans many areas of creative fiction ~ including the very wide romance genre ~ as well as her published non-fiction self-help guides, personal growth and development ebooks, and a large number of articles and posts across the web on a variety of sites and blogs about smart modern shopping, style, music, the arts, and a range of eco-friendly topics. She lives in New England with her *devoted* in their dream home, and they make sure to enjoy the wonderful aspects of life on a daily basis.

Her most recent book is <u>Beginner's Guide to Writing and Self-Publishing Romance eBooks</u>

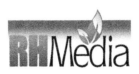